# Limu Moui

## PRIZE SEA PLANT OF TONGA AND THE SOUTH PACIFIC

**Rita Elkins, M.H.**

For order information or other inquiries, please contact us:
Woodland Publishing
P.O. Box 160
Pleasant Grove, Utah
84062
Visit us at our web site: www.woodlandbooks.com
or call us toll-free: (800) 777-2665

ISBN 1-58054-097-X
Printed in the United States of America

# Limu Moui: An Introduction

The unusually low death rate and the high incidence of healthy centenarians (persons over 100 years of age) in Tonga have prompted curious observers to ask, *why*? If you were to query Tongans for possible answers, they would probably refer you to a nondescript sea plant they have harvested and consumed for over 3,000 years. *Limu moui*, a marine vegetable native to their coastal regions, is believed by Tongans to be a source of longevity, health and vigor.

Recent scientific research on limu moui has revealed that the peoples of Tonga have excellent reasons to boast about their brown seaplant. As a natural restorative and rejuvenator, it packs a powerful punch. In fact, it contains a fascinating biochemical called *fucoidan*, which has been compared to human breast milk for its impressive nutrient array. Fucoidan has been the subject of over 300 scientific studies, and it is what makes limu moui so unique. Consider the following:

- Individuals who consume limu moui have increased longevity and disease resistance.
- Limu moui is a highly nutritive sea plant loaded with colloidal minerals gleaned from the ocean itself.
- Limu moui contains fucoidan, a natural substance with antitumor and anticancer properties. It has been compared to mother's milk because of its superb immune support.
- Limu moui is loaded with live plant enzymes that are completely absent from cooked foods. These enzymes boost protein digestion, immune function and overall health.
- Limu moui is rich in *polyphenols*—impressive natural antioxidant compounds that collect dangerous free radicals capable of damaging cells and causing degenerative conditions.

> **FACT:** Limu moui contains a remarkable natural compound called fucoidan that has been compared to breast milk because of its exceptional value to human health and wellness.

Certainly, among an infinite variety of ocean flora, limu moui is one of the most remarkable renewable marine botanicals we have discovered. Relatively unknown and untapped biochemical isolates extracted from limu moui provide us with some of the most impressive nutritive and medicinal substances available, and as a dietary staple, it has provided the people of Tonga with superior nutrition. By contrast, according to some estimates, almost half of the U.S. population is suffering from diseases and ailments (i.e. immune dysfunction, heart disease, diabetes and cancer) related to nutrient deficiencies and poor diet.

## Limu Moui: Health Secret of the South Pacific

In the pristine and unspoiled temperate seawater off the coast of Tonga, limu moui thrives in dense aquatic forests. In fertile, sea-bottom soil, the plant grows creating large ocean meadows of waving angel-like hair. Living in symbiosis with other sea life, limu moui flourishes in virgin Tongan waters. (Not surprisingly, the liquid most like our own life-giving body fluids is seawater.)

In Tonga, local kahunas (medicine men) have long practiced traditional healing methods and have understood well the restorative properties of limu moui, but until recently, the potential of limu moui was unknown in the United States. Relatively undiscovered and untapped by Westerners, limu moui has only been thrust into the spotlight because of the curiosity of health-minded individuals.

Soon, however, questions arose about superior longevity, vigor, disease resistance and overall body strength and stature in Tongan people. Investigations into the routine consumption of limu moui on the islands were initiated, and researchers attributed the resonant health of native Tongans to the unique marine plant.

## What Exactly Is Limu Moui?

Simply stated, limu moui is a member of the brown seaweed family native to Tonga. In fact, the word "limu" means nothing more than "seaweed." Limu moui is also known in other regions as *angel's hair, mozuku* and *nano.*

## WHAT DO THE ANTIOXIDANTS IN LIMU MOUI DO?

- **detoxify the body of heavy metals, free radicals and toxins**
- **improve the structure of hair, skin and nails, and boost their growth**
- **boost gastrointestinal function**
- **reduce high blood sugar and cholesterol levels**
- **protect cells from malignant replication and damage**
- **fight degenerative diseases and aging on a cellular level**

As scientific data on its constituents emerge, this singular ocean organic is creating new interest among biochemists. In its natural edible form, limu moui offers remarkable nutritive, immune-building and disease-fighting properties. As an extract, it promises an even wider variety of therapeutic applications. And for those of us who will probably never cultivate a taste for this extraordinary sea vegetable, its availability in supplemental extract form is good news.

## The Simple Seaweed: Oceanic Wonderfood

Don't be fooled into thinking that seaweeds are just mundane botanicals. These underwater plants are far from ordinary and more than just a diet fad. Compared to ground plant life, seaweeds have remarkable phytonutrient power (phyto means plant). One of the most remarkable of these nutritive plants is brown algae.

Brown algae make up *the largest segment of seaweed plants and include over a thousand species.* South Pacific varieties of brown seaweed can grow up to 213 feet in length. Tongan limu moui grows as part of the vast blanket of marine algae that covers coastal areas around the Tongan islands. As a seaplant, limu moui lacks true stems, leaves and roots, but these hardy plants possess strong structures that provide them with secure

*Investigations into the routine consumption of limu moui on the islands were initiated, and researchers attributed the health of native Tongans to the unique marine plant.*

anchors even in the midst of heavy surf activity. In addition, they can be free-floating plants or grow directly out of the ocean floor.

Typically, limu moui attaches to solid objects and absorbs nutrients directly from the water. (Ocean water contains over seventy-

**WHAT'S SO GREAT ABOUT SEAWEED?**

For thousands of years, seaweeds have been consumed for their exceptional nutrition. In fact, these marvelous plants appear to:
• prolong life
• prevent disease
• significantly enhance health

seven elements.) Because it so readily absorbs compounds in the water, the purity of its environment is crucial. *It can take in toxins, radioactive residues and heavy metals as easily as it does nutrients.* Thankfully, limu moui grows off the shores of Tonga in virgin, unpolluted sea soils at the low-tide mark and creates dense areas of nutrient-rich, uncontaminated underwater vegetation.

In fact, limu moui's natural environment helps make it such a stellar seaweed. In a marvelous symbiotic loop typical of Mother Nature's infinite ingenuity, limu moui gives back more than it takes from its environment.

Since the beginning of time, a variety of shellfish have relied on brown seaweed for their very sustenance. Tongans and other South Pacific locals consider limu moui to be the perfect food—exceptionally well-balanced and sporting an extensive variety of vitamins and minerals (calcium, magnesium, iron, copper, manganese, zinc, boron, iodine), as well as fiber, amino acids and biotin.

## Limu Moui: A Quick Nutrient Breakdown

Limu moui contains a balance of synergistic nutrients *in proportions designed by mother nature.* Below is a list of some of the compounds found in limu moui:

• glyconutrients (galactose, mannose, xylose)
• seventeen amino acids (including glycoproteins)
• a wide range of essential and nonessential fatty acids
• a broad spectrum of essential minerals and vitamins
• a variety of polyphenols (powerful antioxidant plant compounds that protect the body from dangerous free radicals)

> **FACT:** The glyconutrients in limu moui are vital for optimal immune function. Several studies have found that people with unbalanced levels of the eight essential glyconutrients are more likely to have diseases such as anemia, rheumatoid arthritis, respiratory infections and even cancer.

*Limu moui's polyphenol content alone is enough reason to consider it a valuable dietary supplement.* The polyphenols found in limu moui act as superb cell protectors that help prevent:

- malignant growths
- degenerative diseases
- toxic accumulation in tissues
- tissue damage
- skin deterioration

Limu moui possesses other agents that can aid the body in achieving optimal health. These include the following:

- *Fucans and fucoidan*: complex polysaccharides with cancer-protective and immune-stimulant properties, which also raise HGF (hepatic growth factor) for better overall health
- *Organic iodine*: supports normal metabolism and optimal thyroid function
- *Alginate*: a natural detoxifier
- *Laminarin*: an anticlotting and anticancer compound

## Limu Moui: A Storehouse of Natural Minerals

Did you know that you would have to eat dozens of bowls of spinach today to equal the iron content of one bowl served in 1930? This startling statistic is based on a very alarming and widespread phenomenon called soil depletion. Our soils have been stripped of many vital minerals due to modern farming techniques, the use of artificial fertilizers, and fast turnaround harvesting. So that gorgeous head of broccoli or leafy green lettuce may not be supplying your body with the essential minerals it needs to function well and remain disease free.

> **FACT:** Fucoidan and laminarin have been the subject of intensive scientific inquiry and offer dramatic health benefits.

However, in a time when earth's soil may fail to provide us with life-sustaining minerals, we can still turn to fertile seabed plants. In fact, dried brown seaweed has been used as a soil additive to help replenish vital missing minerals.

Limu moui provides an excellent vegetarian source of minerals that has been imprinted with the nutritive content of the sea itself. Seabed soil infuses ocean plants with a vast array of minerals that are in *a natural colloidal form*. Sea "soil" still offers us what we may not be able to obtain from land-grown foods—plants infused with a wide array of colloidal minerals.

## What's So Special about Colloidal Minerals?

- Colloidal minerals retain their integrity even when in a liquid suspension.
- Colloidal minerals are microminerals—their very tiny size makes them much easier to be absorbed through the cell wall.
- Colloidal minerals from plant sources are easily accepted by the body. They are not in a metallic form, which can actually poison the body. Metallic minerals can accumulate in body tissues over time creating organ damage. Overdosing on certain iron supplements can have disastrous results due to this very phenomenon.
- Colloidal minerals make the transport and utilization of other nutrients such as vitamins possible.
- Colloidal minerals facilitate the removal of toxic substances.

Submerged in seawater, the limu moui plant absorbs minerals and vitamins directly from the rich oceanic brew of life-sustaining nutrients. Seawater is rich in minerals such as calcium, magnesium, iron, copper, manganese, boron, zinc and iodine. These minerals are in a colloidal form, making them highly bioavailable. It is also rich in natural vitamins, particularly B1, B2, Niacin, B12, E and biotin. Keep in mind that all the vitamins in the world would render us no health benefits if our bodies are deficient in minerals.

> *Many seaweeds have more vitamin C than fruits like oranges.*

## Traditional Folk Medicine Applications of Seaweed Plants

As mentioned earlier, seaweed has long enjoyed status as a dietary staple in both Asian and Tongan diets. In fact, many seaweeds have more vitamin C than fruits like oranges. And the notion that sea-weeds like limu moui have curative powers for health conditions is nothing new. *Folk practitioners have used these plants to treat cuts, burns, sore throats, allergies, arthritis, bowel disorders, colds, flu, rashes, infections, tuberculosis, parasites, tumors and ulcers.*

Today, the discovery of long-chain or complex polysaccharides in plants like limu moui is thought to explain their extraordinary cura-tive powers. While all of the traditional uses for seaweeds have not been substantiated by medical research, the research that has been done confirms that such underwater plants *offer a myriad of remark-able health benefits.*

Despite these findings, unfortunately, North Americans have had little success cultivating a taste for sea vegetables. For that reason, the notion of using supplements to gain access to their exceptional nutri-tion and health protection is certainly appealing.

## Limu Moui: Asia's Answer for a Long Life

The longevity and good health associated with consuming limu moui is particularly appealing to Westerners. Reports surfacing from certain regions in Japan offer more support for limu moui's potential. In Japan, seaweed dishes such as kombu and wakame are relatively familiar; however, a less-known form called mozuku is used in certain regions of the country. *Interestingly, people native to these regions enjoy exceptional longevity and lower incidences of cancer compared to their other Japanese counterparts.* The inclusion of mozuku as part of a balanced diet is thought to be a major contributing factor to their remarkable health. The same premise applies to the people of Tonga who call the brown sea plant "limu moui."

## Fucoidan: Limu Moui's Secret Weapon

Scientific research into claims about limu moui led researchers to a compound called fucoidan. It is the presence of this unique poly-saccharide (large sugar molecule) in the cell wall of limu moui that makes the sea plant so beneficial for human health. Fucoidan gives limu moui its slippery and somewhat sticky texture, but the protec-tive moisture barrier it provides makes limu moui's survival possible, even when the plant is exposed to strong sunlight.

However, it is the composition of fucoidan that got scientific atten-tion. Fucoidan has a chemical composition that closely resembles one of the most perfect immune-boosting foods on earth—human breast

> ### FUCOIDAN FAMILY HISTORY
>
> There are actually a number of different fucoidans in the fucoidan family. Some scientific studies test only certain classes of fucoidans. These classes include U-fucoidans, F-fucoidans and C-fucoidans. Usually, however, the more general term "fucoidan" is used since distinctions between fucoidans are often minor.

milk. Of equal interest is a tendency of fucoidan molecules to bond with sulphate groups. What does this mean? New studies tell us that the more sulphate groups the plant has, the more therapeutically active it is. Furthermore, limu moui has *one of the highest fucoidan contents* when compared to other marine algae.

## Why Is Fucoidan So Impressive?

The subject of countless scientific studies, fucoidan is clearly one of Mother Nature's most impressive natural compounds. This unique natural plant chemical has been shown to:

- Enhance immunity
- Fight allergies
- Inhibit blood clotting
- Decrease cholesterol levels
- Lower high blood pressure
- Stabilize blood sugar
- Prevent ulcers by fighting *Heliobactor pylori* bacteria
- Relieve stomach disorders
- Improve and support liver function
- Promote hair growth
- Maintain skin moisture and tighten the skin
- Detoxify the body of heavy metals and dangerous chemicals
- Have antiviral, antibacterial and anticancer properties
- Contain powerful antioxidant compounds

## Fucoidan: Essential Immune Booster

Our immune systems are under constant attack and immune disorders are escalating at an alarming rate. New studies are continually emerging that point to immune malfunction as the real cause of conditions like heart disease, obesity and multiple sclerosis. Preventing disease by fine-tuning and supporting our immune systems is the best investment we can make for extended good health and longevity.

Fucoidan's impressive properties make it an excellent supplement for immune support. In fact, scientists have gone so far as to compare its immune boost to that provided by mother's milk. And what could be more supportive to the immune system than mother's milk? Packed with nutrients and antibodies, breast milk helps to arm the naive immune system of an infant with defense cells borrowed from

> *"The composition of the first week of human mother's milk is very similar to fucoidan, which is a major composition of angels hair seaweed [limu moui]. Newborn babies do not have essential antibodies for survival until after the first week, during which time the babies develop an immune system thanks to their mother's milk."*     Dr. Kyosuke Owa

the more experienced immune system of the mother. The fucoidan content of limu moui works much the same way.

According to Dr. Kyosuke Owa, an expert in brown seaweed, fucoidan contains *the same type of antibodies found in human mother's milk*, thereby providing essential nutrients to boost the immune system. Dr. Owa's research findings reveal that fucoidan stimulates the production of vital immune cells, giving the body better armament against potentially deadly invaders—bacteria, viruses, fungi, parasites, and even cancer cells.

## Reinforcing Our Immune Arsenal

The fucoidan in limu moui is not the plant's only immune booster, however. Limu moui contains special sugars called glyconutrients that encourage natural killer (NK) cells to fight diseases of all kinds. Our first line of immune defense is NK cells. Research has shown that when people with poor health increase their consumption of glyconutrients, their natural-killer cell count rises dramatically, making them more able to protect themselves from the tissue breakdown that accompanies degenerative diseases. Limu moui's balanced array of glyconutrients encourages NK-cell and B-cell regeneration, thereby speeding up the body's immune attack against foreign invaders.

In one study conducted at the Department of Agriculture at Kagoshima University, seaweed containing fucoidan was given to mice for twenty days. Upon examination, the natural killer (NK) cells and macrophages (large white blood cells) of test animals had increased to the twice that of the control group.

## Limu Moui Stimulates B-Cell Production

Natural killer (NK) cells aren't the only immune cells affected by limu moui. An article in the March 1997 issue of the *International Journal of Immunopharmacology* reported that seaweed extracts stimulate the production of B cells in the immune system. These cells produce antibodies against the disease organisms we are exposed to and enable our immune defenses to spring into action the moment they are recognized. Researchers in the study also discovered that the glyconutrients of seaweed extract help mobilize white blood cells to better engulf and destroy dangerous infectious microorganisms. They recommended further research on using these sea plants to improve the condition of the immune system.

## Antibiotic Resistance

Limu moui's immune-boosting potential has special meaning for scientists and doctors today because of something called antibiotic resistance. The term refers to smart bacteria that have learned to mutate so as to make themselves impervious to antibiotics like penicillin and its analogs. These super bugs do not respond to traditional drugs and are a growing problem not only in third-world countries, but also in our own hospitals. The causes for this phenomenon are varied, but the results are not—reduced health and even death.

FACT: Cardiovascular disease accounts for almost half of all deaths in the U.S., closely followed by cancer (over a third of deaths) and diabetes (over 10 percent of all deaths).

In fact, the growing number of deaths from these super bugs has prompted organizations like the World Health Organization (WHO) to take action. Still, many believe that antibiotic resistance can only be slowed down, not halted. This reality has prompted a new focus on immune building. If antibiotics fail us, what then? *We must fortify our innate (built-in) defense systems with powerful immune-boosting compounds like fucoidan.*

## Bacterial Infections and Fucoidan

In 1995, European scientists in Romania reported that fucoidan was able to markedly inhibit the growth of gram negative and gram positive bacteria while stimulating the immune system by enhancing phagocytosis (the process of white blood cells engulfing invading microorganisms). These researchers were so impressed with the

> **FACT: In order for our immune system to protect us from infectious and degenerative diseases, we must consume adequate amounts of various glyconutrients. Most Americans consume only one or two types at the most.**

antibacterial action of fucoidan that they suggested further study into the possible use of fucoidan as a drug used to target bacterial infections such as *E coli*.

Furthermore, in a 1995 issue of *Neuroscience Letter,* fucoidan was reported to inhibit the kind of dangerous inflammation that occurs in meningitis (a complication of a bacterial or viral infection). These findings and others show that fucoidan does what no drug can do: fight bacteria while boosting the immune system rather than weakening it.

## Fucoidan for Viral Defense

Perhaps even more exciting than its antibacterial power is fucoidan's potential for fighting viruses like HIV. Fucoidan increases the production of certain types of interleukins and interferons secreted by immune cells (like T cells). In other words, fucoidan boosts the productivity of certain immune fighters. Interleukins and interferons activate different types of immune cells (T cells, NK cells and macrophages) needed to fight infection and sickness. Because of this effect, scientists believe that fucoidan may provide a very effective treatment against the viruses that cause hepatitis, chronic fatigue and even AIDS.

In fact, research data compiled so far suggests that taking fucoidan orally may be beneficial for people who suffer from chronic viral infections such as herpes and cytomegalovirus—a virus that can cause miscarriage and birth defects. Furthermore, fucoidan has been shown to bind to enveloped viruses interfering with their ability to attach to host cells. If a virus can't attach to a host cell, it cannot replicate.

Interestingly, laboratory tests show that the increased production of these immune factors by fucoidan occurs in an antigen-specific way. This means that once certain disease cells are present, fucoidan boosts

> **FACT:** Strep infections are one of the most common bacterial threats facing us today, and they are becoming increasingly difficult to treat due to new antibiotic-resistant strains appearing regularly throughout the world.

the level of immune defense cells *specifically designed to attack those particular invaders*. In this way, fucoidan modulates or enhances immunity when necessary. Because viral infections don't respond to antibiotics, this action is crucial to viral defense.

## Fucoidan and Allergy Prevention

Building our immune system not only helps us fight bacteria and viruses, it also can improve annoying conditions like allergies that are caused by immune system dysfunction. One reason so many people suffer from violent allergic reactions is that their immune systems mistakenly identify substances like pollen, dust and other substances as foreign invaders, and to retaliate, our system produces substances called IgEs that cause sneezing, wheezing, nasal inflammation and other symptoms. IgE is a class of immunoglobulin usually found only in trace amounts in the body and believed to be for parasitic infection; however, allergenic substances can trigger IgE overproduction.

Limu moui may offer allergy relief. The fucoidan content of limu moui provides a balanced nutrient profile that supports *virtually every organ in the body*. Because fucoidan stimulates cell regeneration, it can increase the count of natural killer (NK) cells in the immune system. This action helps boost our ability to fight disease and may also counteract the allergic reactions we see with hay fever and asthma. In fact, some studies out of the Department of Agriculture at Ryukyu University in Japan have found that fucoidan works in several ways to initiate positive immune reactions in the human body. For instance, scientists now know that the fucoidans in limu moui can stimulate the production of interleukin 12 and interferon-fA (proteins secreted by immune cells), resulting in the suppression of IgE overproduction (responsible for many allergy symptoms).

In one experiment, for example, mice were inoculated with a form of albumin that acted as an allergen. Those mice treated with oral supplementation of fucoidans had reduced IgE levels. Consequently, the severity of their allergic reactions was considerably less.

## Fucoidan, Cholesterol and High Blood Pressure

Although fucoidan is known for its immune system benefits, it can have positive effects on other body systems as well. In fact, data from the Laboratory of Lipid Chemistry in Yokohama, Japan, and published in a 1999 issue of the *Journal of Nutrition* reveals that rats fed brown seaweed had significantly lower levels of blood fats than those who were not. After twenty-one days on the seaweed, scientists concluded that brown seaweed compounds alter the activity of enzymes in the liver that control the way fatty acids are metabolized, resulting in lower cholesterol levels in the blood.

Other researchers in Japan conducted a study in which test subjects were given five grams of seaweed (containing fucoidan) per day for three weeks. As a result, their high blood pressure and cholesterol levels significantly improved. Results like these have been reported to the World Health Organization (WHO), and they suggest that the fucoidan content of certain seaplants promotes lipid combustion in the liver—an action that benefits and protects the cardiovascular system. Fucoidan also optimizes levels of HGF (hepatocyte growth factor) in the liver where cholesterol is made and fatty acids synthesized. In addition, there is some evidence that fucoidan may discourage the formation of blood clots, lowering the risk of both heart attack and stroke.

## Fucoidan: Promising Cancer Therapy?

Furthermore, Western science is now supporting the traditional use of limu moui in Asia and the South Pacific to treat cancerous tumors. Data strongly suggests that the fucoidan content of limu moui is the reason why it has shown anticancer potential. More specifically, researchers believe that fucoidan's immune enhancement properties may be related to its beneficial effects on tumors.

## FUCOIDAN'S ANTICLOTTING ACTION

Several research studies have confirmed the ability of fucoidan to discourage blood clot formation. The Department of Surgical Sciences in Stockholm published findings on this matter in a November 2000 issue of the *European Journal of Vascular and Endovascular Surgery*. The scientists concluded, "Fucoidan is a more potent antiproliferative polysulphated polysaccharide than heparin." (Heparin is a prescription blood thinner used to prevent blood clots after surgery.) Swedish doctors at Malmo University Hospital also reported that fucoidan inhibits the formation of blood clots by preventing fibrin compounds from clumping and sticking to artery walls.

In a 1995 issue of *Anticancer Research*, Japanese scientists reported that fucoidan inhibits the spread of lung cancer (metastasis). Using laboratory mice, they found that injections of fucoidan prevented the lung carcinomas (malignant or cancerous tumors) from spreading. They concluded that their findings raise the distinct possibility that fucoidan may have real clinical value in preventing the spread of cancer in the body. Similarly, French scientists discovered the same antitumor effect and refer to fucoidan's "antiproliferative effect" on cancer cells in a 1993 issue of *Anticancer Research*.

## Three Ways Fucoidan Compounds Fight Cancer

1. FUCOIDAN COMPOUNDS ACTUALLY PROMPT CANCER CELLS TO SELF-DESTRUCT. Recent studies reveal that fucoidan compounds actually inhibit abnormal cell growth. Cancer is nothing more than cells that reproduce themselves with no controls. One Japanese study found that when U-fucoidan (one family of fucoidans) was admin-

> *"Results suggest that the antitumor activity of fucoidan is related to the enhancement of immune responses. The present results indicate that fucoidan may open new perspectives in cancer chemotherapy."*　　　*Anticancer Research Nov/Dec 1993*

istered to cancer cells in vitro, they were destroyed within seventy-two hours. The way in which these cells were obliterated is of equal importance. Destruction came from within the cells themselves. Apparently, fucoidan turns on the cellular switch that gets rid of malignant replication. In other words, the DNA found within these individual cancer cells was broken down by enzymes that inhibit the cells themselves. Technically, this is a process called "apoptosis"—a protective mechanism that helps to keep many of us cancer free.

2. ADDITIONAL LABORATORY STUDIES SHOW THAT FUCOIDAN CAN STOP DANGEROUS CELL DIVISION. In tests using human bronchopulmonary carcinoma cells (lung cancer cells), fucoidan effectively blocked the G1 phase of cell division, discouraging the growth of malignant tumors.

3. FUCOIDAN'S IMMUNE ENHANCEMENT PROPERTIES CAN DISCOURAGE CANCER CELL GROWTH. Cancer cells are permitted to replicate because the immune system fails to recognize and destroy them. Fucoidan produces interleukin and interferon compounds in the immune system that inhibit malignant cell growth, thereby having an anticancer effect. In so doing, the effectiveness of natural killer (NK) cells is enhanced, which enables the immune system to destroy malignant cells more efficiently. In light of these

> *Cancer cells are permitted to replicate because the immune system fails to recognize and destroy them.*

actions, fucoidan can play a pivotal role in our immune response to cancer and infection. In fact, it is currently being used for stomach cancer. And in Japanese clinics, it is also being used to treat colon and lung cancer, as well as leukemia. Doctors who use fucoidan supplementation on patients believe it is effective and relatively free of side effects.

Remember also that a breakdown in our immune surveillance system allows cancer cells to grow unrecognized. Fucoidan revs up immune defense cells, and in so doing, they may become more vigilant in targeting abnormal cells for destruction.

## Breast Cancer Prevention with Limu Moui

Japan has one of the lowest rates of breast cancer in the world. Scientists have singled out their consumption of soy as a major contributing factor. But soy may not be the only contributing factor. New data tells us that soy and seaweed could actually work together as a powerful cancer preventive duo. Researchers at the University of South Carolina found that the use of seaweed and soy

> **FACT:** Soy contributes phytoestrogens that can protect breast tissue against exposure to the body's circulating estrogen, which can stimulate the growth of breast tumors.

supplementation in postmenopausal women definitely impacted their hormone levels.

In this test study group, half of whom had been treated for early breast cancer, all twelve women were given a low iodine, brown seaweed supplement for six weeks, and seaweed in combination with a powdered soy supplement. The results strongly suggested a synergistic interaction between the seaweed and soy. Interestingly, the ratio of certain estrogen metabolites excreted in the urine changed from a dangerous to a benign ratio during treatment. This

> *"For cancer to start and then continue growing, it must outmaneuver the many long arms of your immune defenses. The immune system is both your first and last defense against cancer."* John Bailar, M.D., Ph.D., former editor in chief of the JOURNAL OF THE NATIONAL CANCER INSTITUTE

study implies that taking soy and brown seaweed supplements like limu moui together may protect against the formation of malignant breast tumors *in women who have had breast cancer and those who have not.*

## How Does Limu Moui Prevent Breast Cancer?

Limu moui, as a member of the brown seaweed family, works through *six different pathways* to prevent breast cancer. In a report from the Harvard Public School of Health published in *Medical Hypotheses*, scientists suggest that compounds in the plant work to:

- Reduce plasma cholesterol (reduces the risk of certain cancers)
- Reduce the binding of dangerous steroids to breast tissue
- Prevent the transformation of phospholipids to carcinogenic substances
- Inhibit the creation of carcinogenic flora in the bowel
- Protect breast tissue against pollutants and toxins
- Supply vital trace minerals that protect breast tissue

The report points to the routine consumption of brown seaweed by the Japanese *as a significant factor in their unusually low breast cancer rates.*

## Blood Sugar Control with Limu Moui

Limu moui may also offer help for diabetics. In a January issue of *Reproductive Nutrition and Development,* French researchers reported that the polysaccharides found in seaweed positively impacted blood sugar and insulin responses in laboratory animals. The addition of these polysaccharides resulted in what they described as a "dramatically reduced glucose absorption balance." What this suggests is that polysaccharide compounds like fucoidan slow the infusion of glucose into the bloodstream from the intestines, thereby helping to keep blood sugar levels stable and prevent excessive insulin responses. For people with diabetes, insulin resistance or hypoglycemia, this is good news.

## Fucoidan for Stomach Complaints and Ulcers

Limu moui may also be useful for gastrointestinal problems. In several Japanese studies conducted in Tokyo, fucoidan was used in test subjects with routine stomach complaints. Consistent fucoidan supplementation resulted in improved function of the upper gastrointestinal tract. In addition, scientists at the Yakult Central Institute for Microbiological Research recently reported that C-fucoidan prevented the attachment of *H. pylori* (a bacteria that is known to cause gastric ulcers) to cells that comprise the stomach lining. They surmised that this fucoidan compound may have actually coated the surface of the bacteria making it much harder to bind to gastric cells.

## Fucoidan and Stroke Treatment

In 1999, researchers at the University of Manitoba in Winnipeg, Canada, reported that one of the reasons for stroke-induced brain damage is the presence of inflammatory cells. In one study, laboratory rats that experienced a brain hemorrhage were given fucoidan because of its anti-inflammatory properties. Results "showed significantly more rapid improvement of motor function in the first week and better memory retention." This suggests that *repeated doses of fucoidan following a stroke may serve to minimize brain damage and memory impairment.*

**FUCOIDAN FOR JOINTS**

In 1995, scientists discovered that fucoidan helps promote the creation of a substance called fibronectin, which plays a significant role in keeping joints lubricated and flexible. The study found that the presence of fucoidan contributed to the normal production of this substance—a fact which suggests that fucoidan supplementation may be beneficial in cartilage regeneration for arthritic joints.

## Fucoidan Inhibits Peritonitic Inflammation

Fucoidan's anti-inflammatory properties may also help with other inflammatory conditions. Scientists at the Institute of Biomedical Chemistry of the Russian Academy of Medical Sciences in Moscow reported in 1997 that fucoidan can actually inhibit the inflammatory process that contributes to peritonitis (a serious inflammation of the lining of the stomach).

They discovered that the presence of fucoidan prevents inflammation-causing white blood cells from migrating to the site, thereby reducing inflammation. And because inflammatory responses are responsible for many chronic disorders including types of arthritis, allergies and skin disorders, this fucoidan action is very significant.

## Boost Recovery Time with Fucoidan

Fucoidan promotes more rapid recovery of the body because it stimulates better liver cell regeneration (which will be discussed later in more detail). In fact, one study found that oral fucoidan supplementation twice daily in laboratory test animals prompted liver restoration. Healthy liver function helps strengthen the entire body. For people who have been chronically ill, injured in accidents, or have had surgery, fucoidan supplementation may speed up recovery time. Fucoidan not only stimulates tissue replacement in the liver, but in other organs as well—including the skin.

In fact, the combined power of limu moui's colloidal minerals and its fucoidan content help the body cope with stress. The release of cortisol during periods of stress can predispose us to disease by weakening the immune system, but by keeping the body supplied with the restorative compounds and minerals found in limu moui, we provide a shield from the detrimental effects of stress.

# Fucoidan: Skin Friendly from the Inside-Out

As mentioned earlier, fucoidan can stimulate tissue replacement in the skin. In an October 2000 issue of *Biological Pharmacology Bulletin,* Japanese scientists reported that it is the fucoidan content of seaweed that boosts the production of a protein called integrin, which increases skin firmness and repair. The report also emphasized that fucoidan promotes the contraction of collagen gel, which serves to boost wound healing. Other seaweed compounds also serve to fight dryness that can cause premature aging. Seaweed phytochemicals are excellent in topical applications because they often promote the retention of moisture.

In fact, seaweed gel extracts are frequently used in skin emollients and hair preparations. Testing in laboratory animals has shown that the application of brown seaweed extracts (with high levels of fucoidan) for several weeks make the skin more taut. It is also suggested that brown seaweed compounds actually shorten the cycle in which skin cells replace themselves. In so doing, the skin is slower to wrinkle and faster to heal.

Some of limu moui's skin-protecting action may be due to its alginic acid content. Alginic acid helps to keep the plant from drying out due to harsh exposure to the ultraviolet rays of the sun. In fact, limu moui extracts provide an array of compounds ideally suited for cosmetics and hair treatment products of all kinds. For anyone who has lost their hair due to chemotherapy or radiation treatments, fucoidan-containing extracts may be helpful. They can be used both internally and

## LIMU MOUI AND SKIN MOISTURE

As a member of the brown seaweed family, limu moui is high in a substance called mucilage. Mucilage is a gel-like compound that provides protection for delicate membranes and holds in moisture. It can help prevent skin irritation and can contribute to hydration to keep skin flexible and supple. In essence, mucilage can:

• discourage skin dryness

• enhance the absorption of water molecules in the skin

• make the skin more firm and resilient

• boost skin regeneration (for healing and wrinkle prevention)

• strengthen skin, hair and nails

## LIMU MOUI FOR MOOD ENHANCEMENT

It is widely known that people suffering from depression are often low in B vitamins, folic acid, vitamin C, and certain essential fatty acids. Depletion of one of these, DHA (decosahexaenoic acid), is thought to be a major contributing factor to mood disorders. Brown algae contains DHA, suggesting that daily limu moui supplementation may elevate mood.

externally in poultices, gels and compresses. Furthermore, the natural lecithin content of limu moui may help break down fatty deposits under the skin.

## Limu Moui for Appetite and Weight Control

In some European countries, high fiber seaweed is added to foods like bread to create feelings of satiety or fullness. Furthermore, even if the fiber contents of limu moui are removed for liquid extract products, the high mucilage content of the sea plant helps to satisfy hunger.

Moreover, when the right balance of nutrients is supplied to the body on a regular basis, food cravings are often eliminated. Some research has shown that overeating may be due to abnormal food cravings stimulated by nutrient deficiencies or poor carbohydrate or protein food selections. In addition, the iodine content of limu moui can stimulate an underactive thyroid. Underactive thyroid conditions have been linked to slower metabolism and weight gain.

## A Word on Hyperactivity and ADHD

Limu moui may also be helpful for children. Heavy metal accumulation in the body of children may play a significant role in learning disorders and hyperactivity. The amino acids and polyphenols (antioxidants) present in limu moui have the distinct ability to bind to these metals in the urinary tract, thereby keeping them from building up in the bloodstream.

Furthermore, there are almost 6,000 food additives routinely used in foods, many of which have been linked to behavior disorders and allergies. An initial detoxification for any child afflicted with ADHD is recommended as a first step.

# Limu Moui: The Ocean's Fountain of Youth?

Ponce de Leon's legendary search for the fountain of youth may have led him to the ocean. Japanese scientists have discovered that the fucoidan found in limu moui significantly enhances the production of something called IT-IGF or HGF (hepatocyte growth factor). Over the past ten years, Biotechnology Research Laboratories in Japan have been conducting research into the fiber makeup of a several types of seaweed. During the course of these studies, it was discovered that F-fucoidan, found in many brown seaweed plants, can significantly enhance the production of hepatocyte growth factor (HGF).

## What is HGF?

HGF is a very special cytokine that not only stimulates the regeneration of liver cells, but also boosts the production of skin cells, heart muscle cells, cartilage, etc. Investigations reveal that HGF performs a wide array of biochemical functions and is considered vital to the formation of scars and the renewal of organ tissue. We also know that HGF is a protein that slows down the aging process. Several preclinical studies conducted after 1992 have found that HGF can prevent hepatitis, treat cirrhosis, liver failure and pulmonary fibrosis, and slow down the aging process.

One way that HGF treats disease and slows the deterioration associated with aging is by inhibiting a substance in the body that prevents the regeneration of tissue. By so doing, cells replace themselves more efficiently, thereby boosting tissue healing from both disease and injury. This unique therapeutic action suggests that HGF may also be useful in treating challenging degenerative diseases such as diabetes and atherosclerosis.

Japanese studies using lung cells have found that some types of fucoidan react with these cells to boost the production of HGF. In addition, in one study where F-fucoidan was injected into the stomach lining of rats with partial livers, HGF levels were still higher.

The discovery that fucoidan compounds can enhance the production of HGF, not only *holds profound promise for people suffering from liver diseases*, but may also provide hope for all individuals who suffer from degenerative diseases, including the breakdown of tissue that occurs over time as we age.

## Why Do Tongan Seabeds Yield Superior Limu Moui?

Limu moui extracts from Tonga provide some of the purest and most uncontaminated products available. Because Tongan waters are not polluted from industry, supplements derived from Tongan ocean plants are free of the toxins that may exist in the coastal waters around Japan or Europe.

For example, one variety of seaweed commercially harvested off the coast of Wales was abandoned when the threat of industrial pollution from factories and nuclear power plants caused a sharp decline in harvestation.

Furthermore, researchers at the Department of Health Care and Epidemiology at the University of British Columbia in Vancouver, Canada, have issued a report in June 2000 *expressing concern over*

> **FACT: The purity of the water in which seaweed products grow is as crucial as the nutrient profile of the plant itself.**

*radiation and heavy metal contamination of seaweed harvested off the coasts of Japan, Canada and Norway.* They found mercury contamination in six out of eight samples, as well as arsenic residues.

## The Role of Harvesting Methods in the Quality of Limu Moui Products

If possible, using traditional Tongan harvesting practices to collect the plant usually provides the most unspoiled and bioactive product, free of preservatives and toxic residues. Traditionally, Tongans harvest the sea vegetable the same way they have done for centuries, by cutting it away from its fertile seabeds. Any seaweed product should be harvested with care for maximum benefit.

## Limu Moui Extract

While dining on a bowl of limu moui every day would certainly be beneficial, obtaining its nutrient advantage in a supplemental extract form has definite advantages. Even in Asia, the intake of marine sea plants is decreasing, suggesting that dietary supplements may play a profound role in preserving the health benefits of such plants.

Unfortunately, because of its rather unusual taste and texture (a bit rubbery and rigid), the prospect of consistently preparing and eating limu moui is unlikely, to say the least.

Ironically, the alginates, carrageenan, and beta carotene found in brown seaweed are used as stabilizers, thickeners, and food colorants in American foods.

Obtaining the fucoidan found in limu moui through a nutritional product is much more possible and practical. *The accessibility of limu moui in liquid form makes its exceptional bioprotection and support available to people of all ages and cultures.*

Typically, most of us eat on the run and fail to consume the nutrients needed to fuel and maintain a healthy body. Children and the elderly are often malnourished and susceptible to infections and chronic diseases. Various diets and weight-loss plans do not provide a balanced array of nutrients. These and other common scenarios can easily create nutrient deficiencies. Stress, physical demands, surgery, injury or illness demand that we fortify our bodies with supplemental compounds.

## The Advantages of Limu Moui Extract

1. LIMU MOUI EXTRACTS HAVE unique compound profiles that allow the nutrients (in simple cell structure) to be easily assimilated when digested. The molecular weight of the compounds in the extract can be manipulated to make it more bioavialable and concentrated for better therapeutic effect. The indigestible fiber content can be removed to create compounds that are better assimilated for maximum results both internally and externally.

2. THE GLYCONUTRIENTS FOUND in a limu moui extract include mannose, galactose and xylose. The typical American diet contains one or two at the most, and a deficiency of these sugars can cause faulty cell function and transmission, resulting in disease.

3. ESSENTIAL AMINO ACIDS and other vital nutrients are much more concentrated when limu moui is reduced to an extract form.

4. THE COMPREHENSIVE CONTENT of minerals, trace elements, vitamins, amino acids and glyconutrients such as fucoidan are quickly and easily absorbed into the blood stream and through the cell wall much the same way that human breast milk is.

5. THE EASE OF taking a liquid supplement makes it more accessible than consuming limu moui in its whole form.

6. LIMU MOUI EXTRACTS are rich in live enzymes crucial to proper digestion. Cooked foods lack these vital enzymes and put tremendous strain on the digestive system. Bioavailable enzymes found in

> **FACT:** Unlike dried seaweed supplements, limu moui extracts are produced from nutrient-rich portions of the plant. One would have to eat inordinate amounts of limu moui to obtain the high concentration of bioactive compounds in the extract.

limu moui speed the conversion of protein molecules into nutrients that can be readily absorbed and used by the body. By taking an enzyme-rich supplement before eating a meal, we can counteract the ill effects of typical American dietary habits.

7. DOSAGES CAN BE adjusted to increase potency during times of stress or disease.

## Limu Moui Supplements: What To Look For

Look for certified products. Liquid suspensions can include a variety of complementary compounds that carry the limu moui extract itself. Any extract should be produced from pure, fresh, live plants that are carefully harvested and processed quickly without long storage intervals for maximum health and healing benefits. Processing should not use excessive heat, which can breakdown nutrients. In addition, the proper parts of the limu moui plant should be incorporated into the product without the use of chemical pesticide sprays, fungicides or herbicides. Furthermore, care should be taken in order to preserve the alginate and fucoidan content of the plant in extract form. As is the case with all natural supplements, the product should have been tested and bottled properly with labels that include reference material and the manufacturer's guarantee of potency and purity.

# Primary Applications of Limu Moui

| | | |
|---|---|---|
| abrasions | allergies | arthritis |
| atherosclerosis | autoimmune diseases | backaches |
| bladder infections | boils | bowel disorders |
| burns | cancer | chronic fatigue |
| weak circulation | colds and flu | colon diseases |
| congestion | constipation | depression |
| diabetes | earaches | eye inflammations |
| fever | fibromyalgia | gingivitis |
| headaches | heart disease | herpes (cold sores) |
| hypertension | high cholesterol | hyperactivity |
| hypoglycemia | hypothyroid | immune dysfunction |
| indigestion | insomnia | liver disorders |
| menstrual cramps | mood disorders | mouth sores |
| obesity | pain | parasites |
| peritonitis | prostate disease | rashes |
| respiratory infection | sinusitis | skin disorders |
| sore throats | strep infections | stroke |
| toothaches | tumors | ulcers |
| wounds | yeast infections | |

## The Profound Value of Prevention

Unfortunately we live in a disease-oriented society that scrambles to try to treat disease after the fact. Prevention is by far the better way to go and involves the consumption of certain foods and supplements on a daily basis to fortify and protect the body against a whole host of diseases. Using limu moui supplements on a daily basis can do much to prevent illness and give its consumer a much better chance at achieving optimal health and wellness.

# References

Angstwurm, K. et al. "Fucoidin, a polysaccharide inhibiting leukocyte rolling, attenuates inflammatory responses in experimental pneumococcal meningitis in rats" Neuroscience Letter (1995):191:1-4.

Baba, M. et al. "Sulfated polysaccharides are potent and selective inhibitors of various enveloped viruses, including herpes simplex virus, cytomegalovirus, vesicular stomatitis virus, and human immunodeficiency virus" Antimicrobial Agents in Chemotherapy (1988):32:1742-45.

Bartlett, M. et al. "Effects of the anti-inflammatory compounds castanospermine, mannose-6-phosphate and fucoidan on allograft rejection and elicited peritoneal exudates" Immunolgy and Cellular Biology (1994 Oct):72(5):367-74.

Beress, A. et al. "A new procedure for the isolation of anti-HIV compounds (polysaccharides and polyphenols) from the marine alga Fucus vesiculosus" Journal of Natural Products (1993):56:478-88.

Berman, A. et al. "Fucoidan inhibits leukocyte recruitment in a model peritoneal inflammation in rat and blocks interaction of P-selectin with its carbohydrate ligand" Biochemical Molecular Biology International (1997 Oct):43(2):443-51.

Blondin, C. et al. "Inhibition of complement activation by natural sulfated polysaccharides (fucans) from brown seaweed" Journal of Molecular Immunology (1994 Mar):31(4):247-53.

Burton-Wurster, N. "Accumulation of fibronectin in articular cartilage explants cultured with TGF beta 1 and fucoidan" Archival Biochemistry and Biophysics (1995 Jan 10):316(1):452-60.

Chida, K. et al. "Antitumor activity of a crude fucoidan fraction prepared from the roots of kelp (Laminaria species)" Kitasato Arch Exp Med. (1987 Jun):60(1-2):33-9.

Chizhov, A. et al. "A study of fucoidan from the brown seaweed" Carbohydrate Review (1999 Jul 20):320(1-2):108-19.

Colliec, S. et al. "Anticoagulant Properties of a Fucoidan Fraction" Thromb Res (1991):64 (2):143-54.

Criado, M. et al. "Selective interaction of a Fucus vesiculosus lectin-like mucopolysaccharide with several Candida species" Annals of Microbiology (1983):134A:149-154.

Criado, M. et al. "Toxicity of an algal mucopolysaccharide for Escherichia coli and Neisseria meningitidis strains" Rev Esp Fisiol (1984):40:227-30.

Del Bigio, M. et al. "Effect of fucoidan treatment on collagenase-induced intracerebral hemorrhage in rats" Journal of Neurology Res (1999 Jun):21(4):415-9.

Durig, J. et al. "Anticoagulant fucoidan fractions from Fucus vesiculosus induce platelet activation in vitro" Thromb Res (1997):85:479-491.

Ellouali, M. et al. "Antitumor activity of low molecular weight fucans extracted from brown seaweed Ascophyllum nodosum" Anticancer Research (1993 Nov-Dec):13(6A):2011-9.

Fujimura, T. et al. "Fucoidan is the active component of fucus vesiculosus that promotes contraction of fibroblast-populated collagen gels" Biological Pharmacology Bulleton (2000 Oct):23(10):1180-4.

Granert, C. et al. "Inhibition of leukocyte rolling with polysaccharide fucoidin prevents pleocytosis in experimental meningitis in the rabbit" Journal of Clinical Investment (1994):93:929-36.

Heinzelmann, M. et al. "Modulation of lipopolysaccharide-induced monocyte activation by heparin-binding protein and fucoidan" Infectious Immunology (1998 Dec):66(12):5842-7.

Itoh, H. et al. "Immunological analysis of inhibition of lung metastases by fucoidan (GIV-A) prepared from brown seaweed Sargassum thunbergii" Anticancer Research (1995 Sep-Oct):15(5B):1937-47.

Lin, J. et al. "B cell stimulating activity of seaweed extracts" International Journal of Immunopharmacology (1997 Mar):19(3):135-42.

Loenko, N. et al. "Antibacterial and immunomodulating activity of fucoidan" Antibiotic Khimioter (1995 Feb):40(2):9-13.

Maruyama, H. et al. "A study on the anticoagulant and fibrinolytic activities of a crude fucoidan from the edible brown seaweed Laminaria religiosa, with special reference to its inhibitory effect on the growth of sarcoma-180 ascites cells subcutaneously implanted into mice" Kitasato Arch Exp Med (1987 Sep):60(3):105-21.

Millet, J. et al. "Antithrombotic and anticoagulant activities of a low molecular weight fucoidan by the subcutaneous route" Thromb Haemost. (1999 Mar):81(3):391-5.

Murata, M. et al "Hepatic fatty acid oxidation enzyme activities are stimulated in rats fed the brown seaweed" Journal of Nutrition (1999 Jan):29(1):146-51.

Muneer, E. et al. "Mechanism of enhancement by fucoidan and CNBr-fibrinogen digest of the activation of glu-plasminogen by tissue plasminogen activator" European Journal of Drugs and Metabolic Pharmacokinetic (2000 Apr-Jun):25(2):137-43.

Nagaoka, M. et al. "Structural study of fucoidan from Cladosiphon okamuranus" Glycoconutrients Journal (1999 Jan):16(1):19-26.

Newman, B. "Benefits of drinking polyphenols" Optometry (2000 Oct):71(10):619.

Nishino, T. et al. "Effects of a fucoidan on the activation of plasminogen by u-PA and t-PA" Thromb Res (2000 Sep 15):99(6):623-34.

Nishino, T. et al. "Inhibition of the generation of thrombin and factor Xa by a fucoidan from the brown seaweed Ecklonia kurome" Thromb Res (1999 Oct 1):96(1):37-49.

Patankar, M. et al. "A revised structure for fucoidan may explain some of its biological activities" Journal of Biological Chemistry (1993):268:21770-21776.

Pearce-Pratt R, et al. "Sulfated polysaccharides inhibit lymphocyte-to-epithelial transmission of human immunodeficiency virus-1" Biological Reproduction (1996):54:173-82..

Pereira, M. et al. "Structure and Anticoagulant Activity of Sulfated Fucans" Journal of Biological Chemistry (1999): 274: 7656-7667.

Religa, P. et al. "Fucoidan Inhibits Smooth Muscle Cell Proliferation and Reduces Mitogen-activated Protein Kinase Activity" European Journal of Vascular and Endovascular Surgery (2000 Nov):20(5):419-426.

Riou, D. et al. "Antitumor and Antiproliferative Effects of a Fucan extracted from Ascophyllum Nodosum Against a Non-small-cell Broncho-pulmonary Carcinoma Line," Anticancer Research (1996):16(3A):1213-1218.

Shibata, H. et al. "Inhibitory effect of Cladosiphon fucoidan on the adhesion of

Helicobacter pylori to human gastric cells" Journal of Nutritional Science and Vitaminology (1999 Jun):45(3):325-36.

Soeda, S, et al. "A. Fibrinolytic and anticoagulant activities of highly sulfated fucoidan" Biochemical Pharmacology (1992):43:1853-58.

Soeda, S. "Inhibitory effect of oversulfated fucoidan on invasion through reconstituted basement membrane by murine Lewis lung carcinoma" Japanese Journal of Cancer Research (1994 Nov):85(11):1144-50.

Soeda, S. et al. "Oversulfated fucoidan inhibits the basic fibroblast growth factor-induced tube formation by human umbilical vein endothelial cells: its possible mechanism of action." Biochemical Biophysics Acta (2000 Jun 2):1497(1):127-34.

Soeda, S. et al. "Preparation of aminated fucoidan and its evaluation as an antithrombotic and antilipemic agent" Biological Pharmacology Bulleton (1994 Jun):17(6):784-8.

Stein, J. and C. Borden "Causative and beneficial algae in human disease conditions: a review" Phycologia (1984): 23:485-501.

Sugawara, I. "Fucoidan blocks macrophage activation in an inductive phase but promotes macrophage activation in an effector phase" Microbiology and Immunology (1984):28(3):371-7.

Takara Shuzo Co., Ltd. Biomedical Group, Otsu, Shiga, Japan.

Teixeira, M. et al. "The effect of the selectin binding polysaccharide fucoidin on eosinophil recruitment in vivo" British Journal of Pharmacology (1997):120:1059-66.

Thorlacius, H. et al. "The polysaccharide fucoidan inhibits microvascular thrombus formation independently from P- and L-selectin function in vivo" European Journal of Clinical Investment (2000 Sep):30(9):804-10.

van Netten, C. et al. "Elemental and radioactive analysis of commercially available seaweed" Sci Total Environment (2000 Jun 8):255(1-3):169-75.

Vaugelade, P. et al. "Non-starch polysaccharides extracted from seaweed can modulate intestinal absorption of glucose and insulin response in the pig" Reproductive and Nutritional Development (2000 Jan-Feb):40(1):33-47.

Venkateswaran, P. "Interaction of fucoidan from Pelvetia fastigiata with surface antigens of hepatitis B and woodchuck hepatitis viruses" Planta Medica (1989 Jun):55(3):265-70.

Zapopozhets, T. et al. "Antibacterial and immunomodulating activity of fucoidan" Antibiot Khimioter (1995):40:9-13.

Zhuang, C. et al. "Antitumor active fucoidan from the brown seaweed, umitoranoo (Sargassum thunbergii)" Bioscience Biotechnolgy Biochemistry (1995 Apr):59(4):563-7.

# About the Author

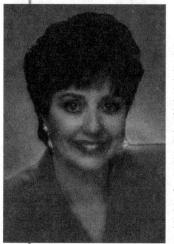

RITA ELKINS, M.H., has worked as an author and research specialist in the health field for the last ten years, and possesses a strong background in both conventional and alternative health therapies. She is the author of numerous books, including *The Complete Home Health Advisor,* which combines standard medical treatments with holistic alternatives for more than 100 diseases, *The Pocket Herbal Reference, The Complete Fiber Fact Book,* and *The Herbal Emergency Guide.* Rita has also authored dozens of booklets exploring the documented value of natural supplements like SAMe, noni, blue-green algae, chitosan, stevia and many more. She received an honorary Master Herbalist Degree from the College of Holistic Health and Healing in 1994.

Rita is frequently consulted for the formulation of herbal blends and has recently joined the 4-Life Research Medical Advisory Board. She is a regular contributor to *Let's Live* and *Great Life* magazines and is a frequent host on radio talk shows exploring natural health topics. She lectures nationwide on the science behind natural compounds and collaborates with medical doctors on various projects. Rita's publications and lectures have been used by companies like Nature's Sunshine, 4-Life Research, Enrich, NuSkin, and Nutraceutical to support the credibility of natural and integrative health therapies. She recently co-authored *Soy Smart Health* with *New York Times'* best-selling author Neil Solomon, M.D.

Rita resides in Utah, is married, and has two daughters and two granddaughters.

# Woodland Health Series

## Definitive Natural Health Information At Your Fingertips!

The Woodland Health Series offers a comprehensive array of single topic booklets, covering subjects from fibromyalgia to green tea to acupressure. If you enjoyed this title, look for other WHS titles at your local health-food store, or contact us. Complete and mail (or fax) us the coupon below and receive the complete Woodland catalog and order form—free!

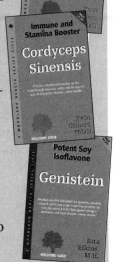

## Or . . .

- Call us toll-free at (800) 777-2665
- Visit our website (www.woodlandpublishing.com)
- Fax the coupon (or other correspondence) to (801) 785-8511